Open, Please!

a Work Book

to Help You Get the Most Benefit from the Text

by

Dr. Kenneth B. Rundle

How to Use This Workbook

Choosing a new dental provider is a complicated task that can result in a happy long-lasting relationship or, if hurried, can result in disaster. Care should be taken in selecting a new dentist to be
sure that your expectations and his are in alignment. If you have dental insurance, you first must decide
if you will restrict your choices to providers who participate in your plan. At times, the level of care you
desire may not be available from a provider who takes your insurance. Dentists are like auto mechanics, lawyers, or any other service provider. There are some great ones, good ones, and some better left alone.
This workbook presents an ordered rational approach to seeking dental care. If this methodology is followed, you should have no trouble finding a provider who satisfies your dental wants and needs. Remember to take advantage of the tips given here and in my book, "Open, Please. A Consumer's Basic Guide to the Practice of Dentistry".

For initial referrals, seek the advice from local pharmacists or practitioners who have been in the area for a good many years. They should not be affiliated with a particular chain of store or hospital group, but independent. Pharmacists associated with a particular chain tend to be relatively new and get shifted around between various store locations so that their knowledge of local providers is fairly scanty. Physicians associated with a particular health or hospital group will usually refer within their network regardless of the individual's overall capabilities when compared with professionals in other groups. A good referral requires the opinion of an individual not beholding to any particular group.

If such independent referrals are not possible, then fall back on the opinions of people you know and trust who have lived in the area for some time. These would be neighbors, friends, co-workers, fellow parishioners, etc.

Take the referrals, go on line and check out the Doctors and offices you have chosen. See the services offered, the office staff, and get a little feel for the corporate culture of the office. Download any forms you might have to complete before you see the dentist to cut down on the time you spend in the reception area and maximize the time available to spend with the dentist and his staff.

If interested, you can also go to the state dental board website to see if any complaints have been filed against the practitioner. Of less relevance, you can also check out the dentist's ratings on Google, Yelp, and the like. These ratings tend to reflect the best and the worst experiences individuals have had and usually do not give you a good overall picture.

Read the associated book, then these suggestions, go forth and find your new dental home. Good luck!

KBR

My Dental Workbook

Let's Analyze Your Smile

Your Name: ____ Date of Birth: _______________

First, find a mirror and stand in front of it. Smile at yourself. Don't be shy. If you are a guy, imagine you are smiling at the most beautiful woman in the world. If you are a gal, imagine you are smiling at the most handsome hunk you can think of.

Look at your smile. Do you like what you see? If the answer is "yes", then go on to Chapter 2. If your answer is "no", then let's analyze why.

A). First look at the teeth themselves. Are they (circle what's appropriate for you):

1. Not white enough
2. Discolored
3. Missing
4. Unevenly spaced (gaps between or overlapping)
5. Crooked, Twisted
6. Broken
7. Worn
8. Mobile (move when you push on them)
9. Painful or tender when biting or closing
10. Surrounded at the gum line by white gook or hard build-up
11. Trapping food in nooks and crannies

B). Look at the gums (again, circle what pertains to you). Are they:

1. Puffy, red, swollen (Do you see pus? Have a bad taste or bad breath?)
2. Bleeding easily
3. Too visible when smiling or not visible when smiling
4. Painful
5. Receding to the point of showing "black triangles" between the teeth

If you circled any of the above conditions, take heart in the knowledge that your dentist can either fix them for you himself or refer you to a specialist who can. But before you go running out to the nearest dental office inquiring about a fix for your peeves, a little home work on your part is required. You will need to gather some information in advance.
Many times, when a patient arrives for a dental appointment for the first time, he or she is presented with a sheaf of papers to complete in a short period of time. Mistakes or forgotten critical information is common when someone is "under the gun" to get the information on paper quickly. Before the patient ever arrives at the office he or she should go online to the office's web site and see if the new patient paperwork is available for downloading. If it is, then a great deal of time can be saved by completing the documentation long before the first visit. This will allow the dentist and staff to spend more time with the patient at the initial visit. If the new patient forms are not immediately available on line, then it is a good idea to write down the information that will be asked in advance so as not to leave out any critical facts. Use the following forms to help provide the complete picture of your medical and dental health.

Correct answers to the following questions will allow your dentist to treat you on a more individual basis, providing the care appropriate for your particular needs.

Name ____ Birth Date _________________________ Age __________

Why are you seeking dental treatment? ____

Please answer each question. Check yes or no. If in doubt, leave blank.   YES   NO

Are you in good health now? ____ ☐ ☐
Are you now under the care of a physician? If yes, what condition is being treated? _________________ ☐ ☐

____

Have you ever been hospitalized or had a serious illness? If yes, explain: ______________________ ☐ ☐
____ Date of last physical exam: ______________
Have you ever had excessive bleeding following an extraction, or do cuts take longer to heal now than previously? __________ ☐ ☐
(Women) Are you pregnant? If yes, what is your due date? ____ ☐ ☐
        Are you nursing? ____ ☐ ☐
Do you use tobacco in any form? If yes, how much? ____ ☐ ☐
Do you have more than two alcoholic beverages per day? ____ ☐ ☐

Do you have now, or have you ever had any of the following?

GENERAL	YES	NO	HEART/BLOOD VESSELS	YES	NO
Tire easily, weakness	☐	☐	Rheumatic fever	☐	☐
Marked weight change (up or down)	☐	☐	Heart murmur	☐	☐
Night sweats	☐	☐	Chest pain/discomfort	☐	☐
Persistent fever	☐	☐	Heart attack/trouble	☐	☐
SKIN			Shortness of breath	☐	☐
Eruptions (rash), hives	☐	☐	Swelling of the ankles	☐	☐
Change in skin color	☐	☐	High blood pressure	☐	☐
EYES			Congenital heart disease	☐	☐
Visual change	☐	☐	Mitral valve prolapse	☐	☐
Glaucoma	☐	☐	Artificial heart valve	☐	☐
EARS			Pacemaker	☐	☐
Loss of hearing	☐	☐	Heart surgery	☐	☐
Ringing in ears	☐	☐	Other	☐	☐
NOSE			**BONE/MUSCLES**		
Frequent nosebleeds	☐	☐	Arthritis	☐	☐
Sinus problems	☐	☐	Artificial joints or limbs	☐	☐
THROAT			**DIGESTIVE SYSTEM**		
Soreness/hoarseness	☐	☐	Hepatitis	☐	☐
NERVOUS SYSTEM			Jaundice	☐	☐
Stroke	☐	☐	Ulcers	☐	☐
Headache	☐	☐	Change in appetite	☐	☐
Convulsions/epilepsy	☐	☐	Black, bloody, or pale stools	☐	☐
Numbness/tingling	☐	☐	**URINARY**		
Dizziness/fainting	☐	☐	Kidney disease	☐	☐
Psychiatric treatment	☐	☐	Increase in frequency of urination (night)	☐	☐
RESPIRATORY			Burning feeling on urination	☐	☐
Tuberculosis	☐	☐	Urethral discharge	☐	☐
Emphysema	☐	☐	Blood in urine	☐	☐
Asthma/hay fever	☐	☐	Venereal disease	☐	☐
Persistent cough	☐	☐	**BLOOD**		
Sputum production (phlegm)	☐	☐	Bruise easily	☐	☐
Cough up blood	☐	☐	Anemia	☐	☐
Difficulty breathing while lying down	☐	☐	Blood transfusion	☐	☐
ENDOCRINE			**OTHER**		
Diabetes	☐	☐	Radiation therapy	☐	☐
Family history of diabetes	☐	☐	Chemotherapy	☐	☐
Thyroid condition	☐	☐	Tumors or growths	☐	☐
Other	☐	☐	Cancer	☐	☐
HIV positive	☐	☐	AIDS	☐	☐

Are you ALLERGIC to or have you ever reacted adversely to any of the following?

	YES	NO		YES	NO
Local anesthetics (novocaine)	☐	☐	Aspirin	☐	☐
Barbiturates/sedatives/sleeping pills	☐	☐	Codeine	☐	☐
Penicillin/other antibiotics	☐	☐	Latex gloves	☐	☐
	☐	☐	Other allergies	☐	☐

Are you now taking any of the following?

	YES	NO		YES	NO
Antibiotics/sulfa drugs	☐	☐	Tranquilizers	☐	☐
Blood thinners	☐	☐	Insulin/other diabetes drugs	☐	☐
Blood pressure medication	☐	☐	Digitalis/other heart medications	☐	☐
Thyroid medicine	☐	☐	Nitroglycerine	☐	☐
Cortisone/steroids	☐	☐	Antihistamines/allergy drugs	☐	☐
Cold remedies	☐	☐	Aspirin	☐	☐
Recreational drugs	☐	☐	Pain medicine	☐	☐
Birth control pills	☐	☐	Other medications	☐	☐
Bone Replacement Drugs for Osteoporosis	☐	☐	Recreational Drugs	☐	☐

If you answered YES to taking any of the above medications, please list the name of the medication and dosage below:

____

____

Is there any other disease, condition, or problem not listed above that we should know about, or is there any activity your doctor says you cannot do? If YES, please explain: _______________________

____

____

____

____

Physician's name ____ Phone ___________________

Address ____

____

Have you ever had any trouble with any previous dental treatment? _________________________________

Does dental treatment make you nervous? (Circle one)   Yes   No   Date of last Dental Visit ___________________

What was done? _______________________   Have you used any dental insurance benefits this year?   Yes   No

Have you ever been treated for gum disease (periodontal disease, pyorrhea)   YES   NO   When? ___________________

Do you now have or have you ever had:

MOUTH	YES	NO	TEETH	YES	NO
Bleeding, sore gums	☐	☐	Loose teeth	☐	☐
Unpleasant taste/bad breath	☐	☐	Sensitive to hot	☐	☐
Burning tongue/lips	☐	☐	Sensitive to cold	☐	☐
Ulcers/fever blisters, lips/mouth	☐	☐	Sensitive to sweets	☐	☐
Swelling, lumps in mouth	☐	☐	Sensitive to biting (pressure)	☐	☐
Braces/orthodontic appliances	☐	☐	Food impaction (getting stuck between)	☐	☐
Biting cheeks/lips	☐	☐	Clenching/grinding	☐	☐
Clicking/popping in jaw	☐	☐	Shifting of teeth	☐	☐
Difficulty opening or closing jaw	☐	☐	Change in bite	☐	☐
Do you snore	☐	☐			

ORAL HYGIENE (DO YOU USE):

	YES	NO
Tooth brush (___ times per day week)	☐	☐
Dental floss (___ times per day week)	☐	☐
Flouride rinse (___ times per day week)	☐	☐
Other	☐	☐

KENNETH B. RUNDLE, DDS
FAMILY & COSMETIC DENTISTRY

Dental Insurance (Benefit) Information You Should Know

(This information is readily available from the insurance representative or HR personnel at the employer's office. It may also be available on the insurance company's website)

Primary Insurance

Insured Name: ____Date of Birth: _______________

Relationship to Patient: self   spouse   child   other

Insured ID or SSN: _______________________________

Employer: ____

Employer Address: ____

    City, State, Zip: ____

    Phone #: _____________________________ Fax #: _________________________________

Insurance Co. Name: ____

Group Plan Name: _______________________________ Effective Coverage Date: ____________

Group Plan #: ______________________________ Insured Member #: _____________________

Member Service Phone #: _______________________________ Fax #: ____________________

Email Address for Claim Submission: ____

Plan Year (Calendar Year or ____________________ to ____________________)

Annual Individual Deductible: $__________________/year

Family Deductible: $________________/year

Annual Benefit: $___________________/year

Amount Used So Far This Year: $____________________

Maximum Age of Dependents for Coverage: _________________

Coverage

In Network - Preventive: ___________% Basic: _____________%

Major: ___________% Perio: ___________%

How Many Quadrants Treatable/Day: ____________/day

Out of Network - Preventive: ___________% Basic: _____________%

Major: ___________% Perio: ___________%

of Fee Schedule: Y   N   or Actual Charges: Y   N

How Many Quadrants Treatable/Day: __________/day

Fluoride: Age Limit: _________ Fee Schedule: Y   N   or Actual Charges: Y   N

Sealants: Y   N   Age Limit: _________ Fee Schedule: Y   N   or Actual Charges: Y   N

Orthodontics: Y   N   Age Limit: _________ Fee Schedule: Y   N   or Actual Charges: Y   N

Dental Implant Coverage: Y   N   ________% Fee Schedule: Y   N   or Actual Charges: Y   N

Frequencies

Exams: _________/year   Healthy Prophy (cleaning): __________/year

Fluoride: __________/year

Replace Lost Sealants: Y   N   Scaling and Root Planing (deep cleaning): ___________________

X-Rays: Panographic Every _______ years   Last Taken: _______________________

Full Mouth Series Every _______years   Last Taken: _______________________

Bitewings (cavity detecting) ________/year   Last Taken: _______________________

Previous Dentist Who Has These Records

Name: ____

Address: ____

City, State, Zip: ____

Office Phone: _______________________________ Office Fax: ____________________________

Crown, Bridge, Denture, or Partial Denture May be Replaced Every ____________ Years.

Other Information

Is There a Missing Tooth Clause (Tooth removed prior to coverage will not be covered by insurance

    if replaced):   Y   N?

Does Insurance Pay Dentist for Services (circle):   As Submitted   Quarterly   Biannually

                                                    Annually

If You Have Another Insurance Plan, Is There Coordination of Benefits: Y   N

Remember, even if you have insurance coverage for a dental procedure, you alone are ultimately responsible for the whole bill. Issues regarding insurance coverage or lack thereof should be worked out before dental treatment begins to avoid unpleasant financial surprises!

Secondary Insurance

Insured Name: ____Date of Birth: ________________

Relationship to Patient: self   spouse   child   other

Insured ID or SSN: _______________________________

Employer: ____

Employer Address: ____

City, State, Zip:____

Phone #: _____________________________________ Fax #: _____________________________________

Insurance Co. Name:

____

Group Plan Name: ____________________________________Effective Coverage Date: ________________

Group Plan #: _________________________________ Insured Member #: _______________________

Member Service Phone #: __________________________________ Fax #: _______________________

Email Address for Claim Submission: ____

Plan Year (Calendar Year or ______________________ to ___________________)

Annual Individual Deductible: $_____________________/year

Family Deductible: $__________________/year

Annual Benefit: $_______________________/year

Amount Used So Far This Year: $_______________________

Maximum Age of Dependents for Coverage: __________________

Coverage

In Network - Preventive: ___________% Basic: _____________% Major: ____________%

       Perio: ___________%

       How Many Quadrants Treatable/Day: _____________/day

Out of Network - Preventive:___________% Basic: _____________% Major: ____________%

       of Fee Schedule: Y   N   or Actual Charges: Y   N   Perio: ___________%

       How Many Quadrants Treatable/Day: __________/day

Fluoride: Age Limit:___________   Fee Schedule: Y   N   or Actual Charges: Y   N

Sealants: Y   N   Age Limit:___________   Fee Schedule: Y   N   or Actual Charges: Y   N

Orthodontics: Y   N   Age Limit:___________   Fee Schedule: Y   N   or Actual Charges: Y   N

Dental Implant Coverage: Y   N   ___________%

Frequencies

Exams: ___________/year   Healthy Prophy (cleaning): ___________/year

                Fluoride: ____________/year

Replace Lost Sealants: Y   N   Scaling and Root Planing (deep cleaning): _______________________
____

X-Rays: Panographic Every _________ years   Last Taken: _______________________________

          Full Mouth Series Every _________years   Last Taken: _______________________________

          Bitewings (cavity detecting) _________/year   Last Taken: _______________________________

Previous Dentist Who Has These Records

          Name: ____

          Address: ____

          City, State, Zip: ____

          Office Phone: _________________________________ Office Fax: ___________________________________

Crown, Bridge, Denture, or Partial Denture May be Replaced Every ____________ Years.

Other Information

Is There a Missing Tooth Clause (Tooth Removed Prior to Coverage Will Not be Covered by Insurance

      If Replaced):   Y   N

Does Insurance Pay Dentist for Services (circle):   As Submitted   Quarterly   Biannually

                                      Annually

If You Have Another Insurance Plan, Is There Coordination of Benefits: Y   N

Other Notes: ____

____

____

____

____

____

Finding the New Dentist

Recommendations of Local Independent Pharmacist (someone who has been in the area for years):

1.   Name: ____

       Address: ____

       City,   State,   Zip:

____

       Office Phone #: ______________________________

       In Network: Y   N   Does he see after-hours emergencies: Y   N   Walk-ins: Y
N

       Hours: Mon________________ Tue ________________Wed ________________

          Thu ________________ Fri ________________ Sat ________________

2.   Name: ____

       Address: ____

       City,   State,   Zip:

____

       Office Phone #: ______________________________

       In Network: Y   N   Does he see after-hours emergencies: Y   N   Walk-ins: Y
N

       Hours: Mon________________ Tue ________________Wed ________________

          Thu ________________ Fri ________________ Sat ________________

3.   Name: ____

       Address: ____

       City,   State,   Zip:

____

       Office Phone #: ______________________________

       In Network: Y   N   Does he see after-hours emergencies: Y   N   Walk-ins: Y
N

Hours: Mon_____________________ Tue _____________________Wed _____________________

Thu _____________________ Fri _____________________ Sat _____________________

Recommendations from neighbors, friends, other employees, fellow church members, other professionals –

4.   Name: ____

Address: ____

City,   State,   Zip:
____

Office Phone #: _________________________________

In Network: Y   N   Does he see after-hours emergencies: Y   N   Walk-ins: Y   N

Hours: Mon_____________________ Tue _____________________Wed _____________________

Thu _____________________ Fri _____________________ Sat _____________________

5.   Name: ____

Address: ____

City,   State,   Zip:
____

Office Phone #: _________________________________

In Network: Y   N   Does he see after-hours emergencies: Y   N   Walk-ins: Y   N

Hours: Mon_____________________ Tue _____________________Wed _____________________

Thu _____________________ Fri _____________________ Sat _____________________

6.   Name: ____

Address: ____

City,   State,   Zip:
____

Office Phone #: ________________________________

In Network: Y   N   Does he see after-hours emergencies: Y   N   Walk-ins: Y   N

Hours: Mon__________________ Tue __________________Wed __________________

Thu __________________ Fri __________________ Sat __________________

Office Contact Check List (1)

Office#: _____ Date Called: _____/_____/__________

Person Answering was:
Slow to Answer	2	3	4	Prompt
Rude	2	3	4	Very Polite
Clueless	2	3	4	Well Informed
Irritated	2	3	4	Eager to Help
Unprofessional	2	3	4	Professional

Person answering identified herself: Y   N   Name: ____

Person answering took relevant information efficiently: Y   N

Person answering gave several appointment options: Y   N

Person answering was able to get you an appointment within a reasonable time period: Y   N

Person answering gave clear and concise directions to the office and materials to bring to your

appointment: Y   N

Other Notes: ____

____

____

____

____

____

Overall first impression: Poor   2   3   4   Great

Office Contact Check List (2)

Office#: _____ Date Called: ____/____/________

Person Answering was: Slow to Answer   2   3   4   Prompt

                           Rude   2   3   4   Very Polite

                           Clueless   2   3   4   Well Informed

                           Irritated   2   3   4   Eager to Help

                           Unprofessional   2   3   4   Professional

Person answering identified herself: Y   N   Name: _________________________________

Person answering took relevant information efficiently: Y   N

Person answering gave several appointment options: Y   N

Person answering was able to get you an appointment within a reasonable time period: Y   N

Person answering gave clear and concise directions to the office and materials to bring to your

                           appointment: Y   N

Other Notes: ____

____

____

____

____

____

Overall first impression: Poor   2   3   4   Great

Office Contact Check List (3)

Office#: ______ Date Called: _____/_____/__________

Person Answering was: Slow to Answer   2   3   4   Prompt

                            Rude   2   3   4   Very Polite

                            Clueless   2   3   4   Well Informed

                            Irritated   2   3   4   Eager to Help

                            Unprofessional   2   3   4   Professional

Person answering identified herself: Y   N   Name: _____________________________________

Person answering took relevant information efficiently: Y   N

Person answering gave several appointment options: Y   N

Person answering was able to get you an appointment within a reasonable time period: Y   N

Person answering gave clear and concise directions to the office and materials to bring to your

                            appointment: Y   N

Other Notes: ____

____

____

____

____

____

Overall first impression: Poor   2   3   4   Great

First Visit Check List (1)

Office name: ____ Dr. Name: ___________________________

Address: ____

Phone: _______________________________   Date visited:___________________________________

First Impression of Office Exterior:

      Neighborhood: Transitional   Urban   Suburban

      Upscale: Yes   No

      Building Exterior: Old   2   3   4   New

                                   Shabby   2   3   4   Well Maintained

      Landscaping: Poorly Maintained   2   3   4   Well Maintained

Upon entering the office, were you greeted by name?   Yes   No

Was the staff member who welcomed you: friendly   neutral   rude?

Is the business office separated from the reception area by: a counter   a sliding glass window?

    (A counter only is an indication of an open friendly office while a closable window indicates a less friendly, more secretive operation).

Was the interior of the office decorated tastefully: Yes   No?

Was there adequate seating available: Yes   No?

Was the seating comfortable: Yes   No?

Was there a selection of current magazines: Yes   No?

Were the magazines neatly displayed and in good condition: Yes   No?

Was water or coffee/tea available to you: Yes   No?

Did you have to wait longer than 15 minutes to be taken back after paperwork completed:

Yes   No?

If you had to wait, was an explanation offered: Yes   No?

Were you escorted back to a treatment room by a staff member: Yes   No?

Was the treatment room clean and inviting: Yes   No?

Were you seated in the room, napkin placed, and the next steps explained to you: Yes   No?

Did the conversations you overheard among the staff professional: Yes   No?

Did the doctor greet you within a reasonable period of time: Yes   No?

Did the doctor seem capable and able to express him/herself clearly and confidently: Yes   No?

Did the doctor go over your health and personal information with you: Yes   No?

Did the doctor prescribe a full mouth series of x-rays and panographic x-ray be taken: Yes   No?

   (A full mouth series of x-rays consists of 18 small films; a panographic x-ray is a whole
   mouth around-the-head picture that shows the supporting bone in greater detail. Both are
   necessary)

Were the films taken digitally (about 1/5 the exposure):   Yes   No?

Was an intra-oral camera used: Yes   No?

Were the films and pictures displayed on a screen in front of you and the results explained by the

     doctor: Yes   No?

Were the instruments used in the exam provided in a sterilization bag: Yes   No?

Did the doctor do a complete examination of the hard and soft tissues of the neck and mouth:

Yes   No?

Were the results entered digitally into an electronic record: Yes   No?

Was an oral cancer screening explained and offered to you: Yes   No?

After the examination, were several treatment options offered to you: Yes   No?

Did the office insurance expert present what the costs of the various options would be: Yes   No?

Were financial options, including third party financing, presented to you: Yes   No?

Once the treatment was decided upon, were the steps to accomplish it laid out clearly: Yes   No?

Were the steps then scheduled to accomplish the treatment: Yes   No?

Overall, did the office environment seem happy and stress free: Yes   No?

Overall, how satisfied were you with the initial visit experience: unhappy   happy   very happy

Other Notes: ____

____

____

____

____

____

First Visit Check List (2)

Office name: _________________________________ Dr. Name: _____________________________

Address: ____

Phone: ___________________________________ Date visited:_____________________________

First Impression of Office Exterior:

      Neighborhood: Transitional   Urban   Suburban

      Upscale: Yes   No

      Building Exterior: Old   2   3   4   New

                             Shabby   2   3   4   Well Maintained

      Landscaping: Poorly Maintained 2   3   4   Well Maintained

Upon entering the office, were you greeted by name?   Yes   No

Was the staff member who welcomed you: friendly   neutral   rude?

Is the business office separated from the reception area by: a counter   a sliding glass window?

     (A counter only is an indication of an open friendly office while a closable window indicates a less friendly, more secretive operation).

Was the interior of the office decorated tastefully: Yes   No?

Was there adequate seating available: Yes   No?

Was the seating comfortable: Yes   No?

Was there a selection of current magazines: Yes   No?

Were the magazines neatly displayed and in good condition: Yes   No?

Was water or coffee/tea available to you: Yes   No?

Did you have to wait longer than 15 minutes to be taken back after paperwork completed:

Yes   No?

If you had to wait, was an explanation offered: Yes   No?

Were you escorted back to a treatment room by a staff member: Yes   No?

Was the treatment room clean and inviting: Yes   No?

Were you seated in the room, napkin placed, and the next steps explained to you: Yes   No?

Did the conversations you overheard among the staff professional: Yes   No?

Did the doctor greet you within a reasonable period of time: Yes   No?

Did the doctor seem capable and able to express him/herself clearly and confidently: Yes   No?

Did the doctor go over your health and personal information with you: Yes   No?

Did the doctor prescribe a full mouth series of x-rays and panographic x-ray be taken: Yes   No?

   (A full mouth series of x-rays consists of 18 small films; a panographic x-ray is a whole mouth around-the-head picture that shows the supporting bone in greater detail. Both are necessary)

Were the films taken digitally (about 1/5 the exposure):   Yes   No?

Was an intra-oral camera used: Yes   No?

Were the films and pictures displayed on a screen in front of you and the results explained by the

   doctor: Yes   No?

Were the instruments used in the exam provided in a sterilization bag: Yes   No?

Did the doctor do a complete examination of the hard and soft tissues of the neck and mouth:

Yes   No?

Were the results entered digitally into an electronic record: Yes   No?

Was an oral cancer screening explained and offered to you: Yes   No?

After the examination, were several treatment options offered to you: Yes   No?

Did the office insurance expert present what the costs of the various options would be: Yes   No?

Were financial options, including third party financing, presented to you: Yes   No?

Once the treatment was decided upon, were the steps to accomplish it laid out clearly: Yes   No?

Were the steps then scheduled to accomplish the treatment: Yes   No?

Overall, did the office environment seem happy and stress free: Yes   No?

Overall, how satisfied were you with the initial visit experience: unhappy   happy   very happy

Other Notes: ____

____

____

____

____

First Visit Check List (3)

Office name: _________________________________ Dr. Name: _________________________

Address: ____

Phone: ___________________________________ Date visited:_________________________________

First Impression of Office Exterior:

Neighborhood:	Transitional		Urban		Suburban
Upscale:	Yes	No			

Building Exterior:	Old	2	3	4	New
	Shabby	2	3	4	Well Maintained
Landscaping:	Poorly Maintained	2	3	4	Well Maintained

Upon entering the office, were you greeted by name?   Yes   No

Was the staff member who welcomed you: friendly   neutral   rude?

Is the business office separated from the reception area by: a counter   a sliding glass window?

(A counter only is an indication of an open friendly office while a closable window indicates a less friendly, more secretive operation).

Was the interior of the office decorated tastefully: Yes   No?

Was there adequate seating available: Yes   No?

Was the seating comfortable: Yes   No?

Was there a selection of current magazines: Yes   No?

Were the magazines neatly displayed and in good condition: Yes   No?

Was water or coffee/tea available to you: Yes   No?

Did you have to wait longer than 15 minutes to be taken back after paperwork completed:

Yes   No?

If you had to wait, was an explanation offered: Yes   No?

Were you escorted back to a treatment room by a staff member: Yes   No?

Was the treatment room clean and inviting: Yes   No?

Were you seated in the room, napkin placed, and the next steps explained to you: Yes   No?

Did the conversations you overheard among the staff professional: Yes   No?

Did the doctor greet you within a reasonable period of time: Yes   No?

Did the doctor seem capable and able to express him/herself clearly and confidently: Yes   No?

Did the doctor go over your health and personal information with you: Yes   No?

Did the doctor prescribe a full mouth series of x-rays and panographic x-ray be taken: Yes   No?

(A full mouth series of x-rays consists of 18 small films; a panographic x-ray is a whole mouth around-the-head picture that shows the supporting bone in greater detail. Both are necessary)

Were the films taken digitally (about 1/5 the exposure):   Yes   No?

Was an intra-oral camera used: Yes   No?

Were the films and pictures displayed on a screen in front of you and the results explained by the

doctor: Yes   No?

Were the instruments used in the exam provided in a sterilization bag: Yes   No?

Did the doctor do a complete examination of the hard and soft tissues of the neck and mouth:

Yes   No?

Were the results entered digitally into an electronic record: Yes   No?

Was an oral cancer screening explained and offered to you: Yes   No?

After the examination, were several treatment options offered to you: Yes   No?

Did the office insurance expert present what the costs of the various options would be: Yes   No?

Were financial options, including third party financing, presented to you: Yes   No?

Once the treatment was decided upon, were the steps to accomplish it laid out clearly: Yes   No?

Were the steps then scheduled to accomplish the treatment: Yes   No?

Overall, did the office environment seem happy and stress free: Yes   No?

Overall, how satisfied were you with the initial visit experience: unhappy   happy   very happy

Other Notes: ____

____

____

____

____

____

        Using the above information, you should now be able to make a sound decision about who you want to place your dental health in the hands of. Enjoy the process; may you have great success!

*"Dentistry is not expensive ---
Neglect is!"*

Anonymous